YES, YOU CAN STOP CITY HALL!

A History of Ambulance Service
in La Crosse, Wisconsin and the
Coulee Region

By David Drewes

AuthorHouse™
1663 Liberty Drive
Bloomington, IN 47403
www.authorhouse.com
Phone: 1-800-839-8640

First published by AuthorHouse 12/2/09

ISBN: 978-1-4490-5650-6 (e)
ISBN: 978-1-4490-5648-3 (sc)

Library of Congress Control Number: 2009912810

Printed in the United States of America
Bloomington, Indiana

This book is printed on acid-free paper.

Table of Contents

Acknowledgements

When I first started this project of researching and writing, I had no idea how many interesting and concerned people I would meet who would contribute in some way to this history of La Crosse ambulance services.

To name a few of the players leaves the possibility of omitting some who deserve recognition, but I will do my best. One of the interesting contacts was former county supervisor Mike Forer who just happened to be in the city when I called his brother to ask about Mike. I learned that Pat Zielke was involved way back in the 60's in a very positive way.

Also to be included are the people associated with Tri-State who were so very helpful but most of all the past director of Tri-State Ambulance, Matt Zavadsky and the current director Tom Tornstrom. Of course, not to be forgotten are the members of our organization, Citizens for Responsible Government, and the 76 circulators of the petition who were critical to the success of the program.

A special thanks goes to Sonja Moe, who helped with grammatical corrections and rewrites. Let me advise anyone who might try a project like this-it is hard work. At the same time if you find someone who is willing to be patient and guide you through the dangling participles or whatever, it can be very rewarding. Also, thanks to my granddaughter Sarah Drewes who provided the initial thoughts for the cover artwork. There are many others who helped me make decisions that, as a new author were quite foreign to me.

While it has been a bigger project than what I had first anticipated, it has been a great pleasure to write this history and especially of the last year's events. I do hope the reader will find it useful as a reference and enjoy the description of how La Crosse, WI, kept a private ambulance service that does not rely on any tax support.

Foreword

The Founding Fathers of our nation were indeed amazing and exceptional people. They were very suspicious concerning the power of federal government and did everything they could to keep political strength divided and at the lowest level possible. The Declaration of Independence is a declaration of freedom from the imperial hand of the King of England. That consideration of the people's right to all our freedoms was strongly argued and is stated in our constitution.

Our early leaders noted that real democracy happens in town meetings where the average citizen has the right to speak, be heard, and possibly have an affect on policy.

Here in La Crosse, there are those who would reduce the number of city council members and county supervisors. They reason that it is difficult to get all the elected fully informed so they might vote knowing the consequences of what is before them. That action reduces responsibility of our elected and is contrary to close representation.

I believe our Founding Fathers would be in favor of having the largest number possible at these levels as this is the first break in the democratic process and begins the republican form of government. Yes, democracy is sometimes messy but it is far and above better than any other known form of government. Benjamin Franklin is quoted, (We have) "a republic, if you can keep it."

It is in this spirit of democracy that Wisconsin has in its constitution the right of its citizens to petition for certain legislation. The Petition for Direct Legislation is only available to Wisconsin citizens due to wise and considerate legislators who wrote this statute so the people of La Crosse were able to make their desires known. Actions in this case under the petition actually required the city to change their plans to take over a private business. Hip, Hip, Hooray!

It is hoped this small book will give inspiration to others who see their local government taking actions beyond what is necessary for governments to do. I am of the belief that local municipalities must keep their eye on the ball and only do what private industry cannot do very well. When there is indicated action that goes beyond that level then it may be time to go to a Petition for Direct Legislation. If that is practiced, then state and federal governments will be kept in check as well.

Dave Drewes

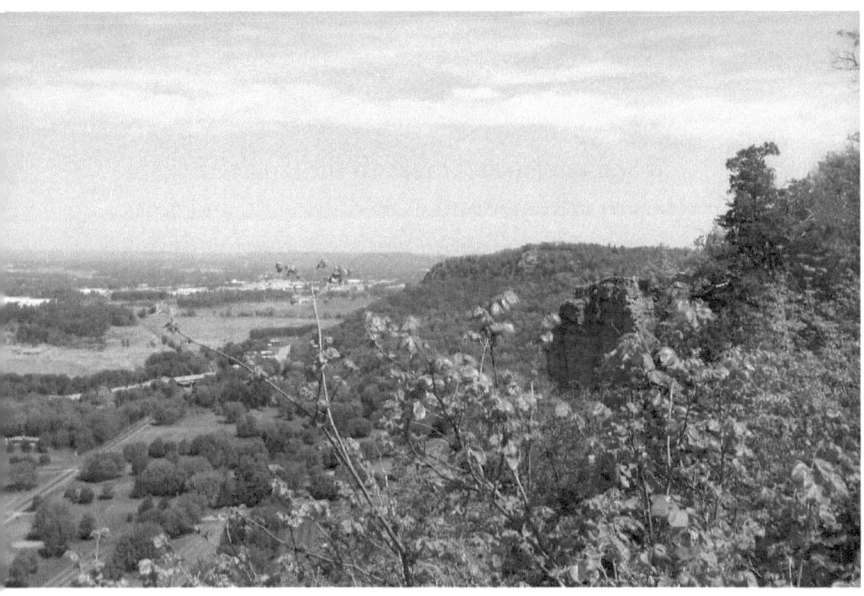

CHAPTER I
The Black Moria and Horizontal Taxis

The history of ambulance service in the county of, and area surrounding La Crosse, is in some ways quite typical and in other ways quite different from those of other smaller market areas. A search for a written history provided some interesting facts, but did not include the developments in 2008 and 2009, so a record of the history including more recent events seemed essential.

The Coulee Region is the name that has been adopted for this beautiful western Wisconsin area. It is descriptive as the area is full of valleys, or coulees as they are known here, cut from the plains surrounding the Mississippi River valley. The remaining bluffs along the Mississippi are as picturesque as any in the country. There are some higher hills that rise above the plain, as this area is a non-glaciated area.

When reference is made to the Coulee Region it refers to extreme southeast Minnesota, and areas north of La Crosse, south along the river, with those areas extending east and west of the Mississippi about 50 miles.

Mr. Ken Jenkerson wrote a paper for the Police Department in May of 2001 that provided some early history of police ambulance services. He noted

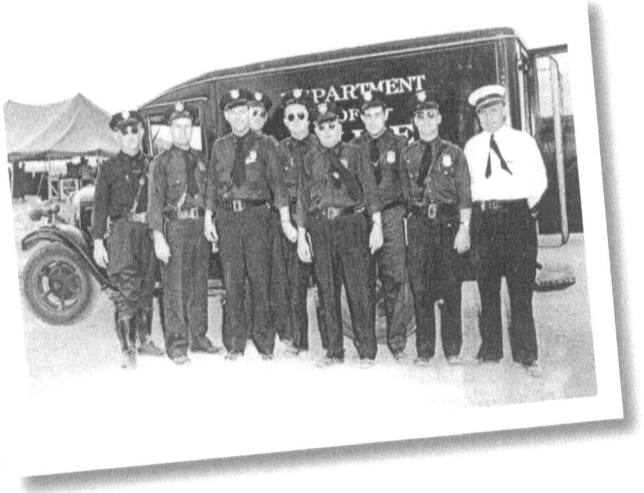

Photo courtesy of the La Crosse Police Department

The photo above is a group of La Crosse Officers posing at the Air Show held in La Crosse on 07-04-46. They are standing in front of the Paddy Wagon called "The Black Maria." From left to right are Ed Miller, Bob Loeffler, R. Thomasguard, Emil Sikorski, John Halverson, Dave Britton, Gordon Engebretson and Aaron Sandford. Photo courtesy Bob Loeffler and Salley Sullivan. La Crosse Tribune.

that until 1946 the city relied upon an aging 1937 Studebaker Ambulance. In 1946 the city purchased a paddy wagon that served a dual purpose as an improvised ambulance as well as police work. It was known as the "Black Maria" (pronounced Moriah). As can be seen it was all black.

In 1949 a Packard ambulance was purchased that

acquired the name "Jet." The Packard was replaced by a Cadillac ambulance in 1962. During this period an ancient Pontiac ambulance was acquired as a backup. To keep the rear door closed they had to put a chain lock on it.

Pat "Doc" Ferguson was head instructor for training for the police force in 1966 as he had been a corpsman in the military. He also was a member of the ambulance crew. Sometimes the police used Harley Davidson motorcycles with a sidecar for transport of accident patients. Non-emergency service was provided in various ways. For a period up until 1960, Dahl Funeral Home provided transport for non-emergencies.

At one time there were five hospitals in La Crosse. (Lutheran, St. Francis, Grandview, St. Anne's, and La Crosse Hospital) The doctors, and possibly others, would transport patients to the hospital. When Grandview, St. Anne's, and La Crosse hospitals consolidated with St. Francis, this service was discontinued. At the same time emergency transportation was provided by the police and sheriff's departments.

Later the vehicles consisted of hearse-style station wagons (also known as horizontal taxis), squad cars, and in some cases private vehicles. These carriers were usually without skilled medical personnel in attendance, and the time of transporting was often critical for survival. By 1968 the police unit had grown to 5 station wagons on the road 7 days a week. The charge per call was $15.00.

As the law-enforcement and fire department

personnel people were only trained in basic survival techniques and were at the scene of an accident or fire to do their work of investigating, fighting fires, and or clearing the scene, proper medical attention was not always available.[1]

Wisconsin recognized the need for higher standards for emergency medical services in smaller communities. The state evaluated local agencies to determine how to improve their operations, and based upon their findings, local law enforcement agencies were ordered to improve their operations.

A true pioneer brings professionalism to La Crosse ambulances

In February of 1968 two sheriff department employees, Herb Garbers and Carl Tabbert, started an ambulance service and called it Tri-State. When it was determined that there was a conflict with their duties as deputies, they sold Tri-State to Walter Gardner. Subsequently, in 1968, a former police officer, Walter "Wally" Gardner took the lead and established this privately run ambulance service for the Coulee Region. He saw the need for better and more professional care in emergency situations. At first, the operation was run from his garage with his wife Joan serving as the dispatcher. Her "office" was their back porch.

This then was the beginning of Tri-State Ambulance, and with it the beginning of modern ambulance service in the La Crosse area.

Wally was a pioneer who aggressively pursued

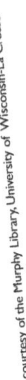

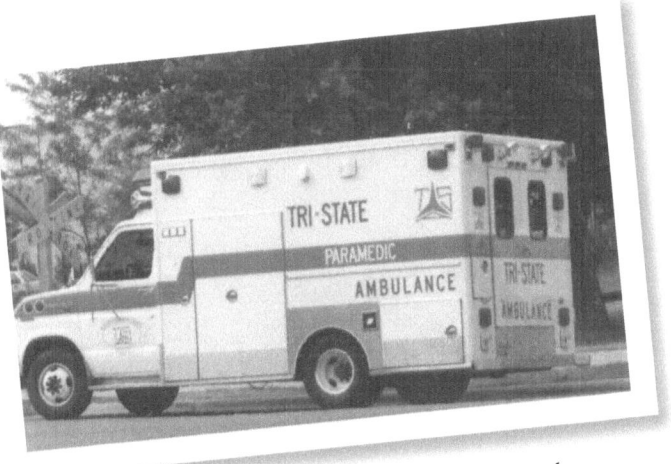

changes
for better medical care en
route to medical facilities. To get more professional
employees, he sponsored several students at
the University of Wisconsin, La Crosse, in an,
"Emergency Medical Technical Training" program.
This innovation eventually led to putting the first
paramedics in emergency vehicles in 1985. In
recognition of his work, Wally was elected President
of the Wisconsin Professional Ambulance Association
in the mid 1980's.[2]

A joint effort of St. Francis and Lutheran
hospitals with Tri-State ambulance established the
"Pre-hospital Advanced Care and Education" (PACE)
program in 1983. The purpose was to provide
standards and procedures for better patient ambulance
care en route to a hospital.

In 1986 PACE contracted with an independent
consultant, "The Fourth Party Inc." to provide
guidance regarding ambulance/paramedic services.
The evaluation authored by Jack Stout, ascertained
the La Crosse market was not big enough to support

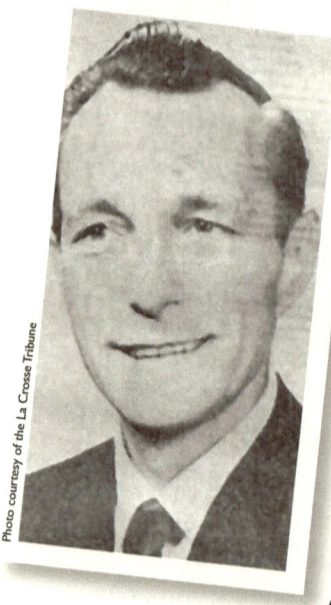
Photo courtesy of the La Crosse Tribune

competing ambulance services without a tax subsidy.

In the mid 1960's alderman Pat Zielke *(pictured at left)* suggested a central emergency communications system, but the idea was not acceptable to the fire, police, or sheriff's departments.

The Coulee Region needed a support system that could coordinate emergency calls from citizens outside the city of La Crosse including the remainder of the county, some Minnesota towns along the river, and other areas just outside the county. The complexity of who should respond, at what level, when, and where needed a plan with structure and coordination. In the early 70's it was recognized that an emergency communications system was essential.

An emergency 911 plan was first considered in 1978. Funding for this project required new radios for all emergency vehicles involved and a dispatch center. A historical event occurred in 1980 when for the first time there was a joint session of the La Crosse aldermen and the La Crosse County supervisors to resolve questions that crossed normal boundary lines.

911 Emergency System becomes a reality in La Crosse

At this time Pat Zielke was the mayor of La Crosse (75-97), and Charles Pierce was the county board chairman (78-85). All forms of funding and other details were eventually resolved, and in January of 1983, a 911 dispatch center became a reality.[3]

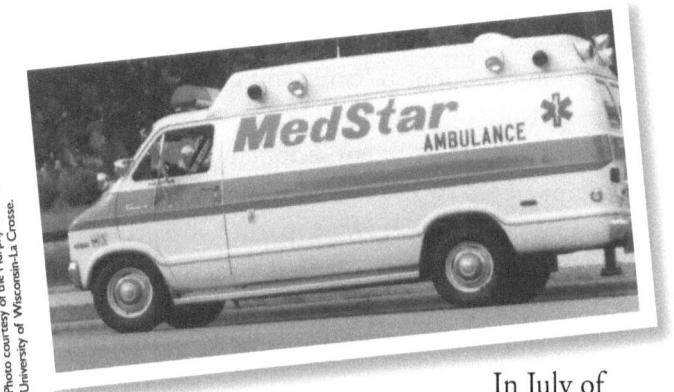

In July of 1985 Steve and Cheryl Paar established MedStar Ambulance Service based in Onalaska. They provided only basic life support for patients, and this limitation caused questions as to whom the dispatcher should be sending on a call. It was difficult for the dispatcher to determine whether paramedic care or just basic care was needed. Both Tri-State and Med-Star questioned the call procedures which determined who was to get which call.[4]

In one instance, the county was sued for not sending Tri-State when a person apparently needed more life support care than MedStar was able to provide. The individual died.[5] The lawsuit was settled in November of 1989.[6]

The La Crosse County supervisors recognized that competing ambulance services threatened the quality of emergency care, and that the conflicts needed resolution. With that in mind, the county law enforcement committee voted to establish an Emergency Medical Services (EMS) board in 1987. This board was to establish criteria for treatment of patients before their admission into a hospital. It would coordinate the 911 dispatch system, law enforcement agencies, and other involved government units.

PACE encouraged formation of the EMS board as the consultant hired by PACE had identified problems with the current ambulance system. Problems noted were poor administration and inadequate equipment. Also, part of the problem, according to the study, was that La Crosse had two competing ambulance companies.

The study, authored by Jack Stout of "The Fourth Party, Inc." recommended the county consider two options:

1. Providing a tax subsidy of $300,000 for non-emergency calls, and

2. having one ambulance service with a monopoly by written contract[7] [8]

Tri-State suffers a great loss

Wally Gardner, (*pictured at right*), died in September 1987 at age 48. He had continued working on improving emergency care and

Photo courtesy of the La Crosse Public Library Archives

pushed for higher standards during his entire career. Former Fire Chief (72-75), Irwin Kahler, noted that he and Wally worked together as a team. When the first responders arrived at the scene before Tri-State, they would stabilize the patients and then turn them over to Tri-State. The actions and cooperation of the first responders continue to be positive today.[9]

Because Mrs. Gardner was very familiar with Tri-State's operation, she continued as owner and operations manager for more than seven years after Wally's death. In 1987 Tri-State had six vehicles and 29 employees. The business was sold to Gundersen Lutheran Hospital in 1995.[10]

The county continued to struggle with the decision of how to resolve the conflicts caused by competing ambulance services. One can appreciate the difficult decisions facing the county supervisors as the problems were serious and needed some governmental attention. At the same time, it was recognized monopolies can be problematic.

Photo courtesy of the La Crosse Tribune

Whatever the action, it would have to be in the interest of high quality care while considering the best method of funding.

Rufus Schmaltz, Greenfield town chair, mentioned that government should stay out of the private business market. "We've got enough government regulation."[11]

In November of 1987 Supervisor Mike Forer, *(pictured above)* chair of the county Emergency

Medical Services Board, said, "By not doing anything, you are telling paramedics they are not wanted in La Crosse County."[12]

People in the area wrote letters to the editor of the La Crosse Tribune asking the county board to make the "right" ambulance decision quickly. Two letters from January 1988 are summarized below:

Robert Kenneth wrote, *Public officials have scrambled to protect their political turf and thus the true issue of comprehensive effective paramedic care has been lost. The issue is quite simple. La Crosse County needs not only to continue providing a system of advanced life support, as it is authorized to do, but also to develop and engage a paramedic service. The resolution by Supervisor Mike Forer represents such a system and deserves attention."*

Julie Schuppel, Franz Fisher, Concerned Citizens for La Crosse County, Paramedic Service Committee, wrote, *"The primary issue is whether La Crosse County will retain paramedic service, not one ambulance service against another or monopoly versus free enterprise. Think about the ones you love and the care you want for them. Please support maintaining paramedic service in La Crosse County, your life may depend on it. Contact Mike Forer, chairman of the Emergency Medical Services board."*

At this time there were four different companies offering ambulance services in La Crosse County. They were, Tri-State, MedStar of Holmen, Quad County Ambulance of Melrose, and Sparta Ambulance.[12]

In January of 1988 the towns of Farmington, Burns and Bangor passed resolutions designating ambulance companies other than Tri-State to be their

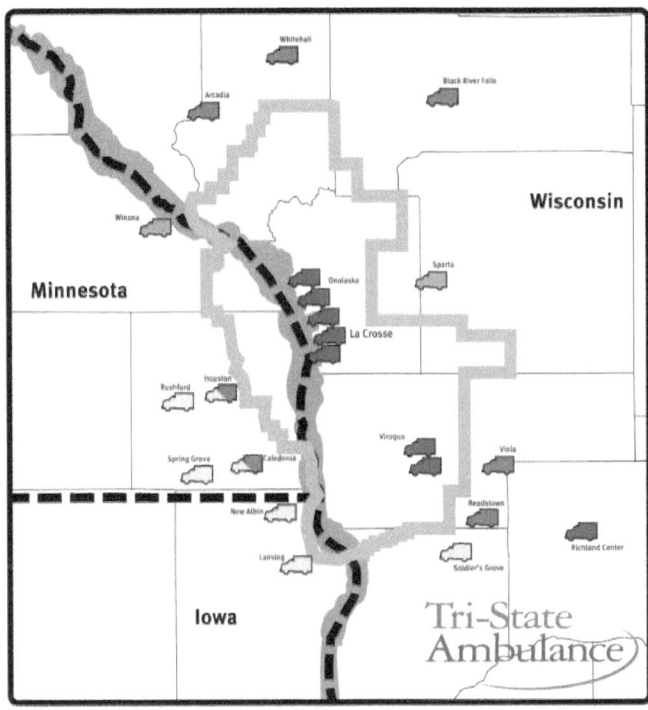

Tri-State's primary service area. Tri-State offers service in nine counties in western Wisconsin and southeast Minnesota.

Tri-State Ambulances:
- 2, Paramedic staffed, 24/7, Hwy 53/OT, Holmen/Onalaska
- 1, Paramedic staffed, 24/7, North Side, La Crosse
- 1, Paramedic staffed, 24/7, South Side, La Crosse
- 1, Paramedic staffed, 24/7, Richland Center
- 1, Paramedic staffed, 12/7
- 1, Paramedic staffed, 24/7, Viroqua
- 1, EMT Intermediate staffed, 24/7, Viroqua

All ambulances are moved throughout the metro La Crosse area based on system status management.

Mutual Aid Relationships:
Tri-State has Mutual Aid agreements with regional ambulances services surrounding its primary service area. The reciprocal arrangement means ambulance services will help one another when needed for back-up.

Mutual Aid Paramedic-staffed Ambulances.

Intercept Agreements:
Tri-State has intercept arrangements with ambulance services in Caledonia, Houston, Spring Grove and Rushford, Minnesota; New Albin and Lansing, Iowa; Soldier's Grove, Wisconsin, as well as other services as needed. The intercept agreement means Tri-State will meet a partner ambulance en route to La Crosse, bringing a higher level of care to the patient sooner.

primary responder. As a result, Tri-State stated that they would no longer be able to provide paramedic staffed ambulances to Farmington, Burns, or Bangor unless specifically requested to do so.[13] The county board passed a resolution in June of 1988 asking that all communities pick a primary and secondary ambulance service by July 15. It required the community have a written mutual aid agreement with a back-up ambulance service.[14]

Another ambulance service, Prehospital Emergency Care Systems (PECS), explored the possibility of beginning area operations in April 1988, however, they discontinued those efforts in June of 1988.[15]

At about this time the La Crosse County Emergency Medical Services Board agreed to work with the two hospitals to formalize an emergency medical care plan. The stated purpose of the plan was to solve the problem of competing ambulance businesses jeopardizing the future of paramedic level care in the area.[16] The Emergency Medical Services Board was formed in 1987 to oversee ambulance services and avoid the need for a county financial subsidy.

Quad-County Ambulance announced plans to end its services in March of 1988. The company had begun operations in 1982 but was plagued by a lack of volunteers.[17] Quad County covered the towns of Farmington, Franklin, Irving, Melrose, and North Bend. Sparta ambulance handled the eastern end of the county while Tri-State and MedStar battled over the central and western parts of the county.

Wisconsin Attorney General James Doyle charged MedStar Ambulance Service, Inc. with defrauding the state's medical assistance program in December of 1994.[18] MedStar ceased operating in 1995.

Tri-State ownership changes

Numerous offers were made to purchase all or part of Tri-State over the years following Wally's death, but Joan wanted to continue the business her husband had started. The battles with competing, but less medically qualified ambulance businesses took their toll and made it difficult to keep Tri-State's operation viable. Finally, in December of 1994, Gundersen Lutheran Hospital announced it intended to purchase Tri-State.[19] Franciscan Skemp hospital declined to be involved in the ownership.

Tri-State was sold as a subsidiary of Lutheran Hospital on March 14, 1995. At this time, some aspects of Tri-State's contract with the county had not been resolved, so the old contract was just extended to December of 1995.

At time of sale Tri-State had 12 ambulances and 70 employees.[20]

There was concern that Tri-State, as a subsidiary of Lutheran Hospital, would not offer the chance for patients to choose which hospital they would be taken to for treatment. It was clarified with a medical control agreement between the two hospitals. This agreement allows full choice by the patient; however, if no hospital was requested, ambulance deliveries would be made to St Francis and/or Lutheran on alternate weeks.

Later studies showed this plan worked very well, and the number of deliveries of patients to each hospital was balanced and equitable.

Thus began a new chapter of ambulance service in La Crosse, La Crosse County, and surrounding communities.

REFERENCES

1   La Crosse Tribune (LCT) 9-15-1987
2   LCT 9-15-1987
3   History of La Crosse Public-Safety Communications Center
4   LCT   9-27-1985
5   LCT 12-11-1987
6   LCT 11-15-1989
7   LCT   8-29-1986
8   LCT   1-13-1987
9   LCT   9-15-1987
10   LCT   3-15-1995
11   LCT 12-22-1987
12   LCT 11-13-1987
12   LCT 11-13-1987
13   LCT   1-26-1988
14   LCT   6-17-1988
15   LCT   6-17-1988
16   LCT   3-16-1988
17   LCT   2-23-1988
18   LCT 12-10-1994
19   LCT 12-14-1994
20   LCT   3-15-1995

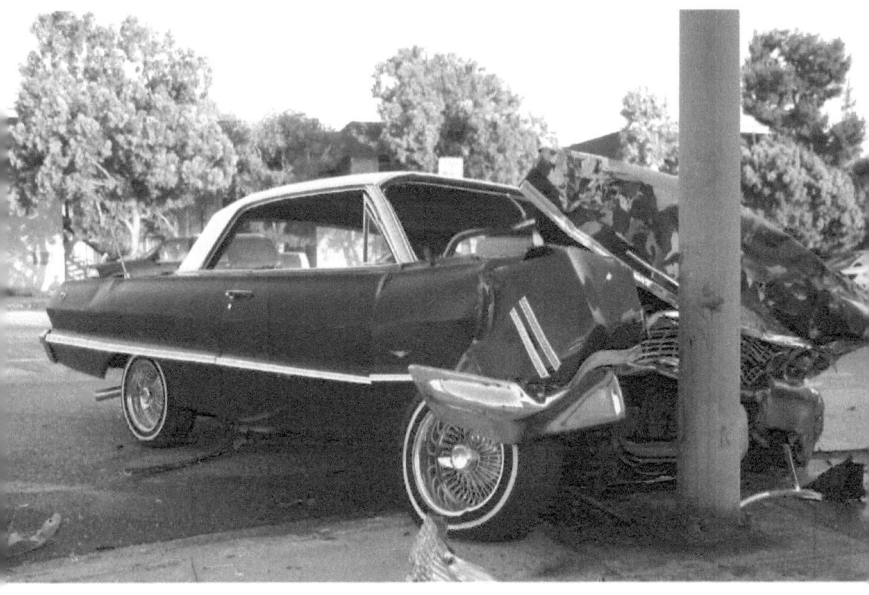

CHAPTER 2
The government monster begins to stir

As ambulance service in the "Coulee Region" evolved over the years from 1968 to 1995, several things became evident. The people of the region recognized the need for high-level emergency medical care, and they wanted it available at their homes or scenes of accidents as quickly as possible. This required thoroughly trained paramedics with fully equipped ambulances on call 24/7.

It also became apparent that standards were necessary to meet the needs of the hospitals and the county residents. The county Emergency Medical Services Board (EMS) found that service was improving. Previous studies and experiences of other smaller markets showed that a community of this size could not support more than one ambulance company unless a tax subsidy was imposed. In addition, without a high number of calls to exercise the required paramedic skills, quality of care would also suffer.

In February of 1996 the Town of Farmington and Tri-State signed a three-year pact that required more of Tri-State than the county contract had. Tri-State was to station an ambulance in Mindoro with Mindoro providing the garage, and that the former Med-Star employees based in Mindoro would be given an opportunity to work for Tri-State. The town was to pay a $75 "no haul" fee when care was given but there was no actual transporting of a patient.

No other support by taxes or other means was to be provided.

Med-Star had received a subsidy of $3,000 annually.[1]

The City of Onalaska had a contract with Tri-State to provide first responder services as well as paramedic care. The fire department was to provide back-up first responder care.

In April of 1998 Onalaska decided their fire department would provide the basic life support first responder service with Tri-State continuing the advanced paramedic ambulance service. Tri-State would no longer keep its ambulance at the National Guard Armory, as the site did not meet Wisconsin State standards for storage. Onalaska felt this new arrangement would better serve its community.[2]

The City looks to expand

In the late summer of 2002 the La Crosse fire department and the city of La Crosse made known their interest in or intention of providing paramedic ambulance services. This was in spite of the history of problems caused by existing multiple ambulance services and the recommendations of consultants who had advised it would cost taxpayers money and that the quality of care would decrease.

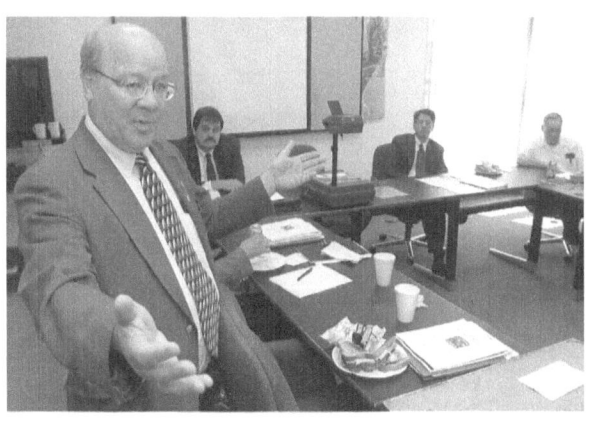

The mayor in 2002 was John Medinger *(pictured above)* and the fire chief was Peter Stinson. However, many La Crosse residents felt that for several years there had been pressure from the fire department to take this action.

At this time, Bernie Mullenbach, city engineer, had stated that the city had gotten out of the ambulance business several years ago and that he wondered why it would want to get into it again. This might have been in reference to the old system in which the sheriff's department and city police did the transporting of patients without good medical supervision such as by a paramedic and/or with inadequately equipped ambulances.[3]

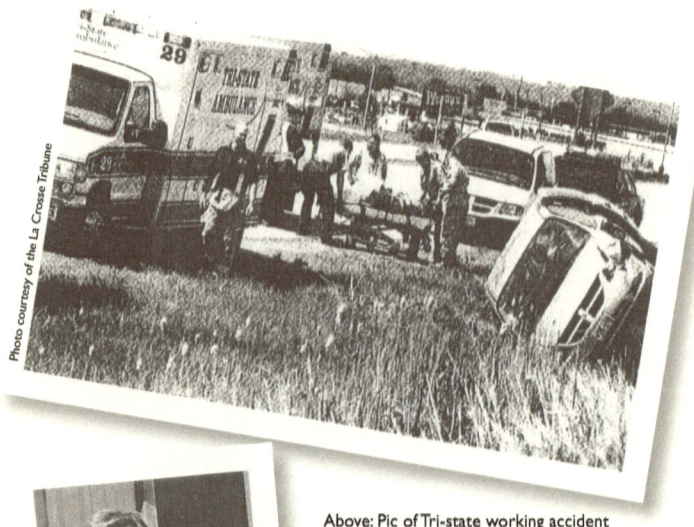

Above: Pic of Tri-state working accident on 5-22-07. Photo courtesy of the La Crosse Tribune. Left: City of La Crosse Mayor Mark Johnsrud

In January of 2006 La Crosse Mayor Johnsrud *(pictured at left)* asked the fire department to update the failed 2002 proposal to have the fire department provide ambulance services. The 2007 capital improvement budget included money for start-up costs. Without a current and realistic analysis of the costs of competing ambulance services, he said he believed it would generate revenue for the city after initial costs were paid.[4]

Fire Chief Pete Stinson was retiring, and the new fire chief would be responsible for carrying out this project. At that time, rumors circulated that the new chief, Gregg Cleveland, was hired having been promised that he would get full backing to get ambulances for the fire department; this would justify hiring more people for the department and a bigger budget. These rumors persisted both locally and in other area fire departments throughout the year of 2008.

Warnings to La Crosse

Statewide, other fire departments had looked at possible financial benefits of providing EMS according to Don Hunjadi, executive director with Wisconsin EMS association. He cautioned that the move would have considerable start-up costs and that none of the last several departments which had considered a similar move had gone beyond the interest and investigation stage; instead they had decided their existing systems were adequate.[5]

In our system of government, it is for all intents and purposes, improper, inadvisable and unethical for any municipal government to compete with private enterprise with any operation that might appear profitable. Governments must be constrained to do only the things that private industry either cannot do or finds impractical.

The county had been involved with concerns about ambulance services for several years; therefore, it was not surprising that in June of 2007 Madison attorney Howard Bellman was hired to act as a mediator to arbitrate the concerns of Tri-State, the city, the two hospitals, and the county.

The initiation of an ambulance service run by the fire department would have a wide spread effect on the county's ambulance costs and the quality of care. It was noted the city's plan differed a great deal from those of the other principals and it seemed impossible to successfully mediate an agreement with the entities involved. Yet, there was hope the mediation might spark some meaningful discussions.[6] (The mediations were to be in closed sessions.)

In an effort to keep the public informed, Tri-State sponsored a forum in June of 2007. This forum was held at the University of Wisconsin La Crosse's Cleary Alumni and Friends Center. One of the speakers was Russ Bayer of Lincoln, NE whose ambulance service was forced to shut down as there was not enough work to support both the city fire department and his business. He warned that the same thing could happen to Tri-State if the city of La Crosse decided to offer the service.

Mr. Bayer also suggested the city's only interests in starting an ambulance service were to employ more city firemen and possibly to generate revenue. He all but blamed the firefighters union for instigating the possible move. Jeff Murphy, head of the local firefighters union objected to the allegation by stating the main goal was for all to work together to improve the system.[7]

There were concerns regarding the closed sessions for mediation. County board chair Steve Doyle justified this strategy by asking the public's indulgence so mediation could go on, "where people aren't beating on their chests or waving flags or whatever, because I think it will be more satisfying of an ending."

Supervisor Medinger was concerned about the proper order of business and raised a point of order to ask, "Doesn't there have to be a proposal on the table?" He was overruled and mediations behind closed doors went ahead with Doyle stating that there would be no secret deal making. All four parties (the city, Tri-State/Lutheran, Franciscan Skemp, and the county) agreed to share in the cost of hiring a mediator, with a limit of $5,000 each.[8]

The mediation efforts with Bellman did not prove fruitful as he did not meet with the four parties after about 6 months or after December of 2007.[9]

An article in the La Crosse Tribune on June 28, 2008 headlines "A year after talks began, mayor hints that La Crosse might soon get its own service." That "hint" implied that the city intended to implement its own plan and was in direct contradiction to Doyle's statement about no secret deal making. In that same article Mayor Johnsrud said, "I think that the county and the city have come to common terms on a plan of action." Hmmm, "no secret deal making?" Doyle did not agree to that so with whom did Johnsrud imagine he had "come to common terms on a plan of action."[10]

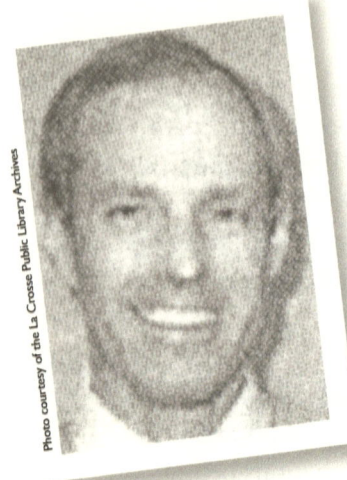

Photo courtesy of the La Crosse Public Library Archives

Matt Zavadsky, *(pictured at left)* director of Tri-State ambulance (06-08) noted one huge benefit resulted from the talks in that an emergency medical dispatch system had been created. However, what agreement had been reached between the city and the county regarding ambulance service was not made public.

A potential closed meeting violation was avoided when some aldermen declined to meet with the mayor and the fire chief. Mayor Johnsrud had asked city council members to meet individually with him and the fire chief to discuss the city's entry into the ambulance business. The meetings were cancelled when the mayor's intention to have the closed meeting became public knowledge.[11]

Total confusion seemed to be reigning in the city and the county as it was noted that, "More than a year of mediation has resulted in a proposal that both city and county representatives have agreed on but that Tri-State 'still has shown reluctance' to sign on to," La Crosse Mayor Mark Johnsrud said. Doyle seems to agree by saying 'the city and county will decide how to go public with details of the proposal.'" [12] If Tri-State had not met with the city and or the county since January, it seemed obvious that they would have "shown reluctance."

Tri-State continued to state that the existing system was functioning exceptionally well, and that fragmentation with the city would threaten the quality and affordability of ambulance services both in the city and in the surrounding areas.

So the controversy finally comes to a head with an announcement that the city and county would release details of a city run ambulance service in a public meeting on the UWL campus on Wednesday August 6, 2008.[13]

REFERENCES

1 LCT 2-14-1996
2 LCT 4-23-1998
3 LCT 7-24-2002
4 LCT 1-28-2006
5 LCT 5-22-2007
6 LCT 6-07-2007
7 LCT 6-21-2007
8 LCT 7-20-2007
9 LCT 7-30-2008
10 LCT 7-30-2008

11 LCT 7-01-2008
12 LCT 7-30-2008
13 LCT 8-02-2008

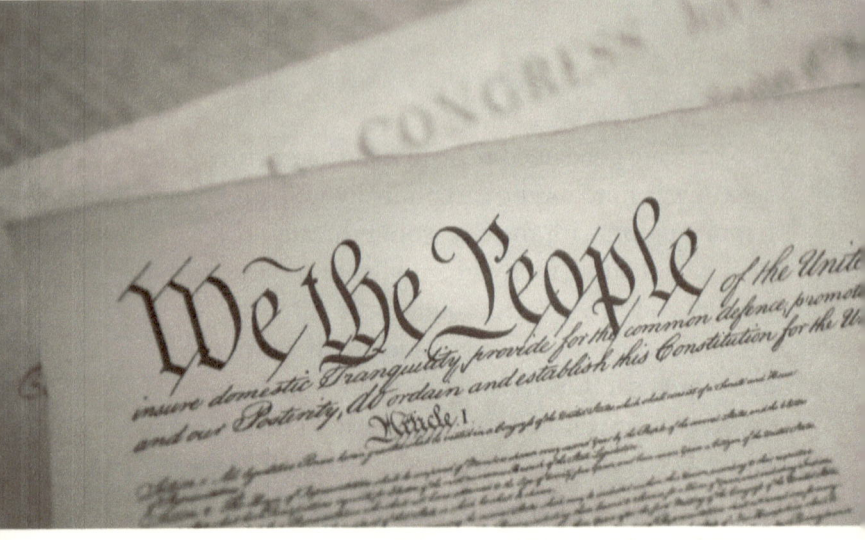

Chapter 3
The Citizens Yell, "NO!"

Citizens for Responsible Government, La Crosse County (CRG), a local watchdog group, was formed in September 2006. It is part of a statewide group headquartered in Milwaukee, is non-partisan, and exposes waste and corruption in local government. While the timing of the founding was during the same year that La Crosse was getting serious about getting into the ambulance business, the group did not have that development on its radar screen at that time. In fact, CRG didn't take an interest in this issue until the summer of 2008.

Members of CRG became more and more concerned about information leaked from the city/county closed meetings. It became obvious that the city, with the fire department, was indeed making detailed plans to establish a city run ambulance system. CRG asked Tri-State to keep them "in the loop" so CRG could do what was necessary to keep the city from expanding into the private sector. Members were concerned for the taxpayers as well as about keeping the existing excellent ambulance service.

In the interest of trying to determine exactly what was being planned and when the closed meetings were to be held by the city and county, open records requests were submitted. The city was very uncooperative only providing one notice of an upcoming meeting but nothing of the past. The county provided copies of a large number of e-mail correspondences.

After more than a year of closed-door meetings with no public input, city and county officials announced they would release details of a municipally run ambulance service on Wednesday, August 6, 2008.[1] That was a shock to many in the city and surrounding areas. State statutes allow closed meetings with very limited exemptions but not for matters of this type.

WI Statute 19.85, Exemptions (e) appears to be the only section which would have allowed Tri-State, the City and County to hold a closed, private session. However, the statute does not mention anything about mediation. A recent court decision of March 8, 2007 by the court of Appeals, in the case of the State of Wisconsin Ex rel Citizens for Responsible Development vs. City of Milton and Milton City Council, reported 2007 WI App 114, 731 N.W.2d 640. This decision shares similarities with the facts concerning the city, county, and Tri-State, and was ruled against the city of Milton, WI.

CRG had become more involved and suggested that its membership attend the August 6th meeting on the UWL campus, Cartwright Building, Valhalla Auditorium. The public needed to be aware that:

1. Tri-State, a private business, operates with no tax money for support.
2. Tri-State has been very efficient and has above average results in patient care and response times.
3. Bigger government invariably means more inefficiencies and higher taxes.
4. The improper, if not illegal, secret closed-door meetings raised many questions about improprieties.
5. There has been no opportunity for public input or debate.

The August 6th meeting called by the city and county was well attended by (approximately 300) city and county residents. The city proposed having one city-owned ambulance by 2010 operating in conjunction with Tri-State. County board chair Doyle clarified that by noting the city would have to purchase two ambulances, with only one in operation at a time and tap new growth in the city rather than erode Tri-States existing business. According to Doyle, the dispatch would send the nearest ambulance to a patient. Johnsrud said the city should recoup its expenses within five years and generate $5,000 in profit.

Anticipating a backlash from skeptical taxpayers present, Johnsrud guaranteed the plan would have no effect on property taxes. Showing disbelief, bits of laughter could be heard from the crowd at this remark by the mayor. An accountant present at the meeting has, as part of his practice, several accounts with ambulance services and concluded the numbers provided by the city were not realistic.

The audience cheered when Steve Gores called on officials to take the proposal to referendum. Johnsrud had been accused of having a tin ear in response to citizens concerns, and this was obvious when he attributed the strong opposition in the audience to those who had ties with Tri-State or Gundersen Lutheran. Refusing to be minimized, unrehearsed, dozens (at least half of the crowd) stood up declaring no such affiliation.

The Emergency Medical Service Commission (EMS) was discussed, and Zavadsky, operations director at Tri-State, called the city's choice of individuals to make up of this commission a deal breaker. Johnsrud got the biggest, incredulous laugh of the night when he said, "People of knowledge shouldn't be the decision-makers on the body."[2] Actually what he was trying to do, was to keep the city in control of the commission and not the county or hospitals.

At this point it should be noted that the mayor's term was to expire in April 2009, preceded by a February primary. He was involved in other controversies, but the primary voter issue would be his stance on a city ambulance service. Eventually, seven candidates entered the primary. The candidates were: Jim Bloedorn, Matt Harter, Mark Johnsrud, Dorothy

Leonard, Mick Lesky, Gary Pedesky, and Andrea Richmond. Most of the candidates were aware of the community's opposition to the city's involvement in ambulance services and either noted opposition to it or were silent on the issue.

Some felt the reason CRG was in opposition to the ambulance plan of the city was to see Johnsrud defeated. That was not the case as CRG was and is primarily an issue-oriented organization. It cares little about who or what party is on the other side of an issue it considers critical. A transcript of an e-mail sent to the mayor by David Drewes CRG local president, on August 7, follows. This e-mail, composed after the disastrous, farcical UWL meeting, makes it quite clear that the issue is the proposal, not the person.

"Mayor Johnsrud, in one short bit of advice to you....Find a way to get out of this mess as quickly as you can. If you didn't know before last night's meeting you surely should know by now that this is a VERY unpopular proposal.

First of all there was nothing provided that would even suggest there was anything wrong with the Tri-State services and secondly nothing was presented that the city would do anything better.

Second, the costs and revenue presented were at best a case of creative bookkeeping. With the firemen average cost being $90,000+ per year and Tri-State's average cost at $60,000+ per year, how can you say that an increase of 50% is not a problem? Further, Tri-State can call in people for partial shifts but give me a clue how the city would do that. If the city would not have to employ more people to run the ambulances then they are about 25 *people overstaffed at this time. Let's save the money and apply it to Bliss road or something that will BENEFIT the people. Maybe reduce taxes rather than find ways to spend more.*

Firemen retire at 55. That means there would be a large turnover and retraining costs associated with new paramedics. Tri-State enjoys dedicated employees for as long as they are capable and want to work.

The city would have to buy two ambulances to cover when one was down for whatever. Was that covered in the cost? Where would they be stored and at what cost?

Other cities have found they must go back to the taxpayers to keep the city run service going. Precisely how would that be different here?

This is a disaster waiting to happen. I do hope that was made a bit clearer to you last night and that you will find a way to quietly drop this crazy idea. From the group that was there, and I believe was quite representative of the population, your future depends on your ability to get this thing killed ASAP."

Dave

Shortly after the August 6th meeting, a letter to the editor read in part, "I decided to go to the meeting since I wanted to learn about the problems with the current system and why the city needed to solve it with its own service. I thought I would hear from the mayor how Tri-State's costs were too high, that they were late on arrival, there was in fighting between the firefighters and Tri-State, or the trucks were zooming through intersections knocking down little old ladies. I found that none of that was true but that the current service ranks as one of the best in the country.

The mayor's reasoning was that if you eat spaghetti all your life, you would have no knowledge of how good steak tastes. I guess his analogy was that his proposal was like steak. Well, when I look at the city's proposal, all I can say is 'Where's the beef?' It looks like the mayor has his meats mixed up, since his proposal looks more like pork to me."[3]

More loss of credibility

The preponderance of opposition somehow impacted the mayor, and he sounded the bugle of retreat, but only half-heartedly, and only temporarily.

On August 14th Mayor Johnsrud introduced a new resolution through council president Bill Harnden. It would create a joint Emergency Medical Service (EMS) Commission but deleted the two city ambulances and training for 12 paramedics who are already employed as firemen.

The key to his new resolution was Johnsrud's statement that, "What we've learned is we need to take this one step at a time." All the resolution did was to remove a timetable for the buying of vehicles and equipment. Council President Harnden said, "If the need were to arise, I think the EMS commission would make that decision." (If the city were to determine the membership of the commission, the group would in all probability include individuals sympathetic to Mayor Johnsrud's agenda.)

Interestingly, the mayor had noted earlier that the city and county were in accord regarding an ambulance commission.[4] That may have been the case but certainly not as to the make-up of that commission.

Council member Bruce Ranis formally requested a public referendum noting, "That cost is way, way, way too much to get into a service that's working well. This is a very foolish idea." His request was voted down.[5]

The county, realizing that the city was changing its position on the EMS, decided it must do something. Doyle said a commission so stacked toward the city "won't fly" in out-county areas. Both the city and county plans have major changes from the plans presented less than 2 weeks ago."[6]

The absurdity went on as the city withdrew its resolution for an EMS commission. "I think there's too many fundamental differences between the city's joint EMS commission compared to the county's," Johnsrud said.

In an almost a side splitting routine, Johnsrud also said that Doyle's plan was a departure from what the camps had agreed upon in months of mediation.[7] Maybe, just maybe, if the city were honest, it would not have continued the delusion about agreements that never were. As Strother Martin's character wryly observed in the film, *Cool Hand Luke*, "What we have here is a failure to communicate." Many thousands of dollars later, the city's representatives were still in denial.

The firefighters decide they must get in on the act, and at a city council meeting spoke in opposition to a public referendum opposing the purchase of ambulance equipment. Dorothy Leonard, who would be a mayoral candidate, said, "I don't want this to be a divisive issue in our community, and that's why I don't support the referendum." She changed her mind when it finally became obvious to her that this was indeed a campaign issue that was going to destroy the candidacy of anyone who opposed it.

David Beach spoke in favor of the ballot item, and scoffed at the implication made by fireman Mike Jorgenson that, " 'The people in this community are not smart enough to make the decisions.' To say we don't know what we're doing is insulting." [8]

CRG members met numerous times to theorize about likely actions the city might take and to discuss how to proceed with a binding resolution. By mid to late September it became obvious, "The city is persisting, and it's working toward giving no indication they're backing away from a city-run ambulance," said Dave Drewes head of CRG. As the city has the ability to start the service if it wishes; a referendum may be the only way for the voters of the city to act to prevent the city's action.

A city-run service would disrupt the entire EMS system for residents of the city, the county and neighboring communities Tri-State now serves.[9]

The Journal of Emergency Medical Services (JEMS), February 2008, reported on a 200-city survey. It is their desire that instead of just reporting data as they have been over the last 25 years, that they would highlight what would be ideal and redirect attention to the potential of EMS.

Some of the highlights noted are:

1. "Government agency operating budgets have almost $3 for every $1 a of non-governmental agency budget."

2. "There's an 18.3% increase in tax subsidy for governmental agencies and a 7.2% decrease for non-governmental agencies in comparison with last year's data."

3. The Journal goes into great detail regarding response times. They are measured in various ways, and if the data is not properly used, erroneous conclusions will be drawn.

That problem developed in La Crosse when Tri-State and the Fire Department used different methods to determine response times. Probably without being aware of the standards, methods used by the local Fire Department favored them rather than using the standards established by industry.[10]

Direct Legislation – True Democracy in Action

At this time CRG established the wording needed for the, "Petition For Direct Legislation" as allowed under Wisconsin state statues. The wording is:

"Be it resolved that the City of La Crosse shall not enter into, nor participate in the formation of, the business or operation of ambulance services."

Formal announcement of the petition was made on October 14, 2008. Jim Bloedorn, city council member and mayoral candidate, was the first to sign the petition at the news conference held at City Hall. CRG would have 60 days to collect a minimum of 2,930 signatures. (15% of voters in the last gubernatorial election)[11]

When an adequate number of city residents' signatures were collected, (CRG plans to get 3,500), the city would verify those as potential voters and present the approved list to the council. The council, at this point, would have only two options, to accept the petitioners' wishes or to put the petition on the ballot at the next regularly scheduled election.

At first our slogan was "If it ain't broke don't fix it;" but it soon became "If it ain't broke don't break it."

REFERENCES

1 LCT 8-02-2008
2 LCT 8-07-2008
3 LCT 8-17-2008 Ltrs to the editor D. Schmidt
4 LCT 7-30-2008
5 LCT 8-15-2008
6 LCT 8-18-2008
7 LCT 8-30-2008
8 LCT 9 -3- 2008
9 LCT 9-22-2008
10 Journal of Emergency Medical Services February 2008
11 LCT 10-15-2008

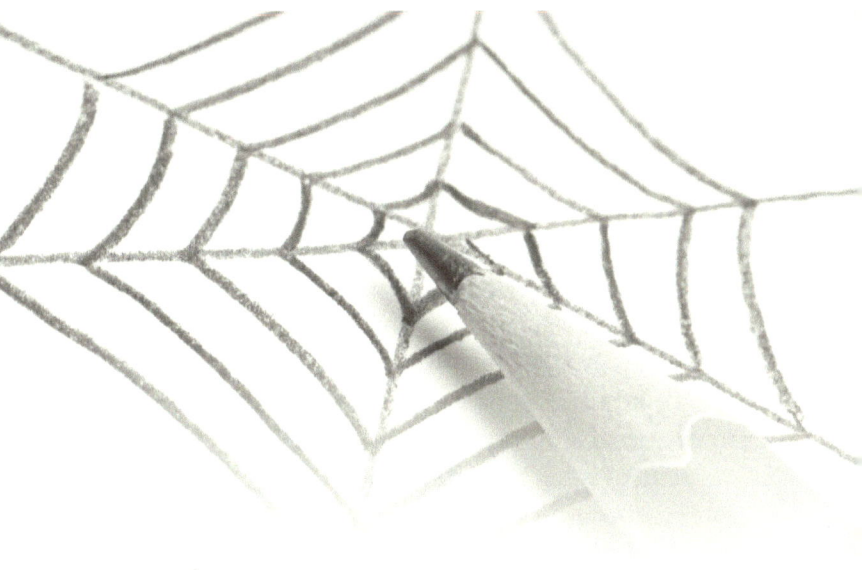

CHAPTER 4
Oh what a tangled web we weave…

Ongoing actions of CRG made the city aware the group was serious about collecting signatures to get the petition certified by the voters. It was also aware that the public was not pleased with the city ambulance proposal and so it began its games to stop CRG's effort even before our October 14, 2008 public announcement.

Council President Harnden announced on October 11 that a new EMS fact-finding commission would be proposed.

The dark little secret was that the plan called for the commission to submit a report to the full council by March. The proposal would restrict the council from taking any action concerning emergency medical services until that report was in hand.[1]

Apparently the mayor, city attorney, and Harden formulated this plan thinking they could stifle the petition drive. Supporters of Tri-State saw through this façade and were energized by this poorly camouflaged parliamentary move.

It was also an obvious move by the city to bypass the county as after many months of "closed-door mediations", Johnsrud continued to say there was agreement when there never was. His ego (or binding promise to the fireman's union) was such that he felt he could confuse the council into doing something that was sure to fail.

The state statute is quite protective of citizens' rights when the correct procedures are followed. In this case, the city's actions were not of consequence, and if they would have been were much too late. A study would only obfuscate the desires of the voters, which are protected.

The job of getting a minimum of 2,930 signatures needed some organization and ideas from our basic core group. We met several times to encourage each other and look for ways to be effective and efficient in getting signatures. We found that some people would volunteer to work their block, just their family, or their friends at work, while others spent many hours at ball games, in front of the post office, or wherever people congregated.

Andrea Richmond was able to secure the use of Roosevelt School for an informational meeting on Wednesday October 22. The public was invited, and a fair crowd was in attendance, including a number of firemen. Upon request, Tri-State made a presentation and then entertained questions. Many people who were there stated they were very satisfied with the service that Tri-State had provided to themselves, their family, or a friend. More than one commentated they would not be at the meeting if it hadn't been for the prompt and excellent care provided by Tri-State.[2]

The firemen were not so pleased as they felt they should have had a place on the program. At that time, it seemed they would be presenting a program to promote their position; also which their presentation would be open to the public. However, that never happened.[3]

Just the facts ma'am, just the facts... Sgt. Friday

Earlier reference was made to the statistics of response time and other factors involved in measuring the effectiveness of ambulance services and that were often misunderstood or misused. The fire department (FD) published a position paper on their web site in October during the time we were collecting signatures. A part of Tri-State's (TS) reply follows:[4]

1. FD says TS's response time was over the target of 7 minutes 54 seconds 90% of the time. TS replied, noting the opposite was true as TS responded to 90% of calls in the city within or under the target time. In fact, TS arrives simultaneously with or before the La Crosse FD nearly 47% of the time. Some of the calls were of non-emergency transports, which means TS travels without lights or sirens.

2. A Milwaukee study showed that when the number of paramedics went up the technical skills decreased. That is a concern in La Crosse if the FD added paramedics. A number of doctors and nurses from La Crosse confirmed that was likely to happen here.

3. TS paramedics have achieved triple the national average for cardiac arrest survival in the city of La Crosse as they feature dual paramedics on all ambulances. TS's average urban call time is 5 min 20 seconds.

4. The above records were achieved with NO taxpayer dollars.

Cost accounting is done in various ways by different municipalities in Wisconsin. In the case of ambulance services, some cities consider some firemen to be in the fire department budget even though they work as paramedics. On the surface that would not seem to make any difference. However, let's look at this a bit more closely.

In the previous notes, TS has been able to attain very positive results, as they are totally dedicated to patient care. If firemen were needed at the fire or accident scene, they would not be totally dedicated to the patient. If, on the other hand, they do dedicate personnel to solely respond to ambulance calls as TS currently does, then these firemen would not be available to respond to fire calls. If they are not available to respond to fire calls, their entire costs must be fully allocated to the provision of ambulance services.

Personnel Cost Example:
FTE's needed for Single Ambulance Staffing   8
    (2 people, 3 shifts, plus 2 vacations, training etc.)
Cost to city per FTE $90,000.
Personnel cost per ambulance $720,000.

    The city has estimated the net revenue for ambulance service will be $337,000, making a loss of $383,000 per year.

    If the city can dedicate 8 firefighters to ambulance service and remove them from other duties without hiring any additional people, it would be much more cost effective to reduce FD personnel by attrition of the eight and save $720,000 per year.

    The elephant in the room then, is the question, is the fire department overstaffed for current duties and if so, by how many?

    The following information from the Sheboygan area is included to indicate how creative a municipality can be if it is determined that a project is to be hidden:

September 21, 2009

Mayor Ryan, Members of the Council and Citizens:

    Last week I obtained a copy of the Fire Department-Ambulance Service Financial & Activity Report for 2008. Some months ago it was reported that the ambulance service made a "profit" of $406,188. This, of course, was computed using only marginal costs and does not reflect all the costs involved in providing this service.

So, **in the interests of transparency,** when one does a full cost analysis and figures personnel costs for 19 paramedics rather than just the four new hires, **the "profit" becomes a deficit of $975,796.**

That figure is even larger when one considers that the information presented in the report does not include any administrative expenses, not one dime for training, although $2,000 was budgeted, and not one dime for the vehicle/equipment lease, which was budgeted at $90,000. Adding the $92,000, one arrives at a deficit of $1,067,796, and we still have not included any administrative costs.

I haven't asked, so I do not know, how start-up costs are being accounted for or repaid, but would, I presume, be an additional expense adding to the deficit.

And the deficit will grow even larger in 2009 when one considers, as discussed at the Finance Committee meeting on August 24th, that both runs and collections were down in the first six months of 2009. **Personnel costs will grow by 10.5% in 2009** because of the pay and bonus increases outlined in the Memorandum of Agreement. Paramedic/firefighters received a 3% pay increase on January 1, 2009, a 1.5% increase on July 1 and up to 24 paramedics received a 3% bonus on January 1, 2009 and will receive an additional 3% bonus on December 31 for a total of 10.5%.

Also of interest is the fact that overtime was 53% over budget and gasoline costs were 101% over budget. Runs and transports exceeded projections by 35%, which accounts for some of this overage. But you have heard me speak before about observing ambulances "tooling" around town and down by the Lake, and I have spoken with numerous citizens on the north and south sides of town who have observed the same thing.

The ambulance drivers evidently are not bothered by wasting gasoline, and they also, obviously, have time to waste. Either neither Chief Lastusky nor any elected official is telling them to stop this practice or they are not following orders.

It is interesting to know that the City of Fond du Lac separates the costs involved in providing ambulance services from their fire department services. At the August 24th Finance Committee meeting, Ald. Bohren stated that **Fond du Lac figured a loss of $1,500,000 for 2008.** They attribute **50% of administrative costs to each service; 75% of paramedic/firefighter personnel costs and 10% of all firefighter personnel costs are attributed to the ambulance service. One would hope that this Council would choose to follow Fond du Lac's model, but, unfortunately, I think that you prefer to see things through rose-colored glasses.**

Moving on to another topic. While I applaud the goals and objectives of the "2010 City of Sheboygan Budget Resolution" which will be discussed tomorrow evening at the Committee of the Whole, I am curious about one of the Whereas clauses, specifically the one that reads: "…..Mid-year impact negotiations requesting the return of a 1.5% July 1st raise failed to get any labor support, thus putting the 2010 budget in further jeopardy." I have been told that the Public Works Union was willing to give up their July 1st 1.5% pay increase and agree to co-payments for their health insurance in an effort to prevent layoffs, but that the City turned it down and instead chose to lay off people.

I was at the Salaries and Grievances Committee meeting on August 24th when the issue was raised, and a DPW spokesperson said that a meeting scheduled for 5:30 that day had been cancelled by the City. I e-mailed Ald. Bouck and Ald. Gischia on September 2nd asking them if DPW had agreed to give up the 1.5% pay increase and agreed to co-payments on their health insurance. Ald. Bouck responded on September 3rd that Ald. Gischia was not on the "labor negotiations team", that I had received "less than half the story", and that the issue was "better explained over the phone". I am still waiting for Ald. Bouck to call me and explain the "rest of the story".

The public has a right to know. Former Mayor Suscha spoke a couple weeks ago about problems the SCTA was having in getting information. Ald. Bohren, Ald. Gischia and Ald. Kliejunas are always very thorough in answering my questions and concerns, but sometimes it seems that some elected representatives **and department heads** do not recognize the public's right to know. I am concerned when there seems to be an effort to withhold information to avoid, I believe, being subjected to further questions or criticism.

Recently I heard either the Mayor or an Alderman talk about the need for transparency. I hope that will be the reality going forward.
Dolcye Johnson
1306 North 3rd Street
Sheboygan WI 53081

Signature gathering on Election Day

With the general election coming up on Tuesday, November 4th it was decided that it would be an excellent time to allow people who were particularly interested in political activities to sign the petition. The petition had to be signed by residents of the city, and this would guarantee that requirement.

We investigated the possibility of being near the polling places, and with counsel, found the following in the Wis. Statutes:

12.03   *(2) (a) 1. No person may engage in electioneering during the polling hours on election day at a polling place.*
(2) (b) 1. No person may engage in electioneering during polling hours on any public property on election day within 100 feet of an entrance to a building containing a polling place.
(4) In this section "electioneering" means any activity which is intended to influence voting at an election.

However, The State of Wisconsin \ Elections Board provided an opinion EL. Bd. 07-01 on March 14, 2007 regarding petitions at or near a polling place as follows:

The Elections Board finds that solicitation of signatures, on a petition that is not related to the election at hand, without any attempt to influence that day's vote of the voter solicited, is not, per se, "electioneering" within the meaning of ss.12.03 and 12.035, Stats, and, therefore, not a violation of those statutes. Further, -circulating a petition within 100 feet of the entrance to a polling place, per se, would NOT constitute a violation of 12.035, Stats.
Also, it is noted that, Mindful that interference with the orderly conduct of the election is a category of conduct wholly separate from "electioneering" and that both interference and electioneering have to be evaluated, in the first instance, by the inspectors at the polling place....

With that opinion, teams were set to be at various polling places. They were advised that while they could be within 100 feet of the polling place entrance they could not interfere with people as they came to vote.

City Attorney Matty either didn't read the law or was highly encouraged to take actions to slow or disrupt the petitioners as they gathered signatures. District Attorney Tim Gruenke correctly noted the ambulance issue was not on the ballot and, therefore no problem existed.[5]

Harassment of the petition circulators by the city started early and occurred often at the polling places.

Examples:

At Altra Credit Union.

City Attorney Matty did admit he was at Altra but denied he did anything to stop efforts to collect signatures. He said he just asked two men to move back at least 100 feet because poll workers said the men were impeding people's right to vote.[5]

Nick Eastman wrote a letter to the editor that said in part, *"While collecting signatures at Altra, the La Crosse City Attorney and an assistant approached us with digital cameras and began taking photographs of the circulators and our signs. I did not recognize the two at first and asked why they were snapping the photos. The city attorney's assistant answered 'You're on public property aren't you?' After recognizing the attorney, I followed up by asking if there was a problem and if we needed to leave. Neither person so much as looked at me. It is of great importance that I emphasize we did not promote or discuss any issues or candidates in this election. We also took great care in assuring we did not interfere with the ability to enter and exit the polling location. I feel very strongly that the administration of the City of La Crosse orchestrated an intimidation campaign to prevent circulators from collecting signatures."* Nick went on to say the two walked right by us after taking the photos without saying a word. After a while they came back out with the election official who said, "I didn't even know they were out here." Matty claimed in a Tribune article on the 5th that poll workers had complained about us.

Jim Yowell's experience

"While at the polling place on the North Side the day of the election, I was asked by two people who did not identify themselves, to move from the front of the polling place. I think I was 100 feet from the door but moved to the northeast corner of the lot, which was, in my opinion, in excess of 100' from the door.

Then another couple, again not identified, told me to get across the street. I could see a large homemade sign on the door of the North side of the building noting this was an exit only. I did move across the street from this door for the rest of the time. Later, a police officer came by and I told him what had happened. He checked with the polling place and returned to tell me I was fine. Looking back, I have the following observations. The person in charge of the polling place never came out to talk to me. It seems to me that people in charge of a polling place should know the law. To me, the unidentified individuals appeared to be politically motivated."

I, Dave Drewes, was assigned to Hintgen School, a polling place on the south side of La Crosse. Upon observation of the entrance sidewalks to the door, I established my sign and material at a point that could be seen from all points but on the grass so I would not interfere with any voters. Just before 4 p.m. a fire and rescue truck with two firemen stopped about a half block south of the school. They got out and stood by their truck. I did not notice if they did anything else as I was busy collecting signatures.

Some days later I was visiting with the Fire Chief, Gregg Cleveland, and I complained about the situation. He said they do inspections of various places and apparently that is what they were doing. I report - you decide.

Shortly thereafter, at 4:06 p.m. by police records,

three squads and, I believe, a fourth car arrived. It made a rather interesting and amusing parade. An officer, Dittman, came and requested I move further away from the entrance. I did so out of respect for him, but I did tell him he had the wrong information about our signature collection. Shortly thereafter, his supervisor came and visited with me stating they were required to have me move. We had a respectful conversation but again I did tell him that they were given bad information.

Not long after that, the city clerk, Teri Lehrke, came to my location to tell me she had complaints in other areas, and she had to enforce the 100 foot rule at all polling locations. I told her she had the wrong information but again did not move back to my original spot as I was collecting signatures the entire time and felt there was no need to challenge the officials who took issue with my location. She did provide me with an e-mail time dated November 4, 2008 at 9:38 AM that was sent to various people, who had apparently complained. It properly noted that the municipal clerk and election inspectors have absolute control of all problems at the polling place; but it went on to say, therefore the 100 foot rule applied, which was in error.

On November 10th WIZM, a local radio station did a short story concerning the events of election day and suggested the city used, "heavy handedness," in opposing the referendum at the polls. Scott Robert Shaw suggested the mayor may have been involved. Well, duh.

The La Crosse common council voted to create

a fact-finding commission as proposed by council president Harnden on November 13, 2008. This resolution, in conflict with the provisions of the state statute, again made the proviso that no action was to be taken by the council until March when the fact-finding commission study was to be complete.

City Attorney Matty apparently approved this measure, either based on his misunderstanding of the law or under pressure from the mayor.

CRG called a news conference on November 24th to present approximately 3,900 signatures to the city clerk.

This was an amazing accomplishment as it only took 40 days to get these signatures. CRG thanked the 76 circulators who spent untold hours getting those signatures.

Victory seemed near when on December 9, 2008, City Clerk, Teri Lehrke, certified 3,436 names as valid for the petition:

Be it resolved that the City of La Crosse shall not enter into, now participate in the formation of, the business or operation of ambulance services.

REFERENCES

1 LCT 10-11-2008
2 LCT letter to ed 10-24-2008.
3 LCT guest ed 10-28-2008
4 TS memo to city council 10-27-2008
5 LCT 11-5-2008
5 LCT 11-5-2008

I, the undersigned, a qualified elector of the city of La Crosse, request that the below proposed resolution, without alteration, either be adopted by the Common Council, or referred to a vote of the electors pursuant to the provisions of S. 9.20, Wis. Stats.

"Be it resolved that the City of La Crosse shall not enter into, nor participate in the formation of, the business or operation of ambulance services."

SIGNATURES OF ELECTORS	STREET & NUMBER OR RURAL ROUTE Rural address must also include box or fire no.	POST OFFICE ADDRESS WHEN DIFFERENT THAN MUNICIPALITY IS NOT SUFFICIENT. THE NAME OF THE MUNICIPALITY OF RESIDENCE MUST ALWAYS BE LISTED.	
		MUNICIPALITY OF RESIDENCE Indicate City or Village	DATE OF SIGNING
1.	314 5 9th St		
2. Andrea Richmond	1312 Cameron Run St.	LaCrosse	10/14/08
3.	710 So 16th Street	La Crosse	10/14/08
4.	314	La Crosse	10/14/08
5.			
6.			
7.	1919 S		

CERTIFICATE BY CITY CLERK
OF PETITIONS SUBMITTED REGARDING
CITY AMBULANCE SERVICE

STATE OF WISCONSIN)
COUNTY OF LA CROSSE) SS.
CITY OF LA CROSSE)

I, Teri Lehrke, hereby certify that I am the duly elected and acting Clerk of the City of La Crosse, Wisconsin, and as such official, I further certify that attached hereto is a true copy of a petition requesting that the following resolution be adopted by the Common Council, or be submitted to a vote of the electors of the City of La Crosse:

Be it resolved that the City of La Crosse shall not enter into, nor participate in the formation of, the business or operation of ambulance services.

I further certify that I have carefully examined said petition and find the same to be in proper form, and that it is sufficient in all respects under the provisions of Section 9.20 of the Wisconsin Statutes.

I further certify that the total number of valid signatures appearing on said petitions is 3,436.

I further certify that the number of signatures needed is 2,930, which is 15 percent of the votes cast for governor at the last election held in November 2006, with 19,535 votes being cast.

In testimony whereof, I have hereunto set my hand and the official seal of the City of La Crosse this 9th day of December, 2008.

Teri Lehrke, City Clerk

**Victory seemed near when on December 9, 2008,
City Clerk, Teri Lehrke, certified 3,436 names as valid for the petition.**

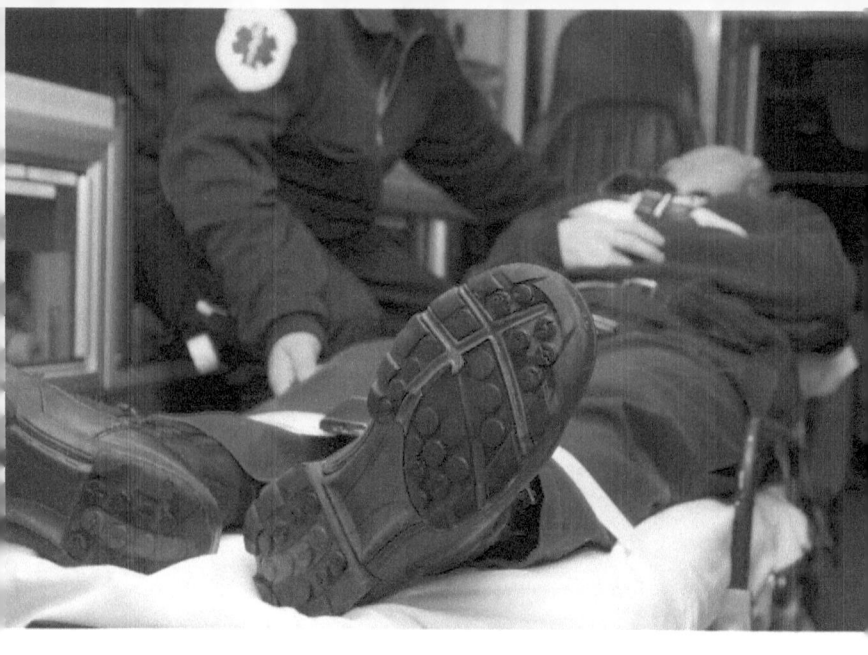

CHAPTER 5
Victory in spite of City Attorney's opinion

The city continued to do whatever it could to confuse the public in general and the Common Council in particular.

To review, CRG started the petition drive on October 14, 2008. As the city was well aware we were about to circulate the petition; on October 10, 2008 Council President Harnden proposed a fact-finding commission. The study part of the proposal was fine; however, the part that declared no action was to be taken regarding ambulance services by the Fire Department until March, was totally out of order, as that would be in conflict with state statutes. Obviously, if that were legal, any direct legislation could be stopped by continual studies. The proposal was approved by the council on November 13, 2008 but had no effect on the petition drive.

At this point I want to emphasize I am not an attorney, however, with counsel it is not that hard to read the law.

City Attorney Matty wrote an error filled Legal Memorandum on 12-9-2008. The conclusion of Mr Matty's report reads as follows:

For the reasons stated above, the proposed resolution submitted through Wis. Stat. ~9.20 would substantially repeal or amend Resolution # 2008-11-013. Accordingly, the Common Council may decide (1) to take no further action and not place the proposed resolution on the ballot; (2) to place the proposed resolution on the ballot for advisory purposes only; (3) to adopt the proposed resolution with alterations consistent with Resolution #2008-11-013; or (4) to reconsider Resolution #2008-11-013.

This conclusion is in direct conflict with the Wisconsin statutes which take great care to protect the voters when a petition is properly drafted and presented. The petition had been carefully reviewed prior to publication and had met all the requirements of the law. The memorandum caused the council to waste many hours debating the subject.

The following contains excerpts from a paper in "The Municipality" September 1991 by Curtis A. Witynski, Assistant Legal Council.

Electors in Wisconsin cities and villages are authorized to initiate ordinances and resolutions using the direct legislation procedures described in sec. 9.20,

Stats. (Section 9.20 was amended by 1989 Wisconsin 273, effective May 4, 1990, to allow electors in villages to initiate ordinances and resolutions.)

Section 9.20 provides that a number of electors equal to at least 15% of the votes cast for governor in the last general election may file a petition with the municipal clerk requesting that an attached ordinance or resolution (hereafter "ordinance"), **without alteration,** (emphasis mine) either be adopted by the governing body or referred to a vote of the electors. Sec. 9.20(1).

Once a petition is filed, no name may be removed. In addition, no signature may be counted as valid unless the date of the signature is less than 60 days before the petition is filed. Sec. 9.20(2m).

Clerk's Role: Within 15 days after the petition is filed, the clerk must determine whether the petition is sufficient and whether the proposed ordinance is in proper form. The clerk must state the findings in a signed and dated certificate attached to the petition. If the petition is found insufficient or the proposed ordinance is not in proper form, the clerk must "give the particulars, stating the insufficiency or improper form." Sec. 9.20(3). The petition may be amended by petitioners to correct any insufficiency or the proposed ordinance may be put in proper form within 10 days following affixing of the clerk's certificate and notification to the petitioners.

When the original or amended petition is found sufficient and the original or amended ordinance is in proper form, the clerk must so state on an attached certificate and immediately forward it to the governing body. Sec 9.20(3).

Governing Body's Role: The common council or village board **must, without alteration, either pass the ordinance within 30 days following the date of the clerk's final certificate, or submit it to the electors for a vote. Sec 9.20** (4). (*emphasis mine.*)

A governing body has no authority to make an initial judgment regarding the constitutionality of an ordinance submitted by the electors under sec. 9.20 unless the unconstitutionality is clear from prior adjudications on the same subject manner.

Therefore, 'a proposition of unresolved constitutionality must be placed on the ballot even though its constitutionality is in substantial doubt.' State ex rel. Althouse v. City of Madison Wis, 79 Wis.2d 97, 255 N.W. 2d 449, 455 (1977).

Scheduling the Referendum: If the governing body chooses to submit the proposed ordinance to the electors for a vote, the referendum must take place at the next spring or general election, if the election is more than 6 weeks after the date of the governing body's action on the petition or the expiration of the 30-day period whichever first occurs.

The ordinance need not be printed in its entirety on the ballot, but a concise statement or its nature must be printed together with a question permitting a voter to indicate approval or disapproval of its adoption. Sec 9.20(6).

City ordinances adopted pursuant to sec. 9.20 are not subject to the veto power of the mayor. City or village ordinances adopted pursuant to sec. 9.20 may not be repealed or amended within 2 years of adoption except by the vote of the electors.

Limitations on Direct Legislation

Although sec. 9.20(4) provides that a municipal governing body must, when presented with a sufficient petition for direct legislation, either adopt the attached legislation within 30 days or submit it to a vote of the electors, the courts have "carved out certain exceptions which indicate that, under some circumstances, the…. [governing body] ….may properly refuse to accept either of the statutory choices and may instead reject both of them." *Althouse*, supra, 255 N. W. 2d at 453 (1977).

The courts have recognized the following five limitations on direct legislation under sec. 9.20:

1. *Administrative in Character.* The ordinance sought to be passed must be legislative in character.

    Proposed legislation which is administrative in character is not a proper subject of initiative proceedings. Althouse, supra, 255 N. W. 2d at 453-54.

    It has been said that actions "relating to subjects of permanent and general character are usually regarded as legislative, and those providing for subjects of temporary and special character are regarded as administrative….." In addition: 'The power to be exercised is legislative in its nature if it prescribes a new policy or plan; whereas it is administrative in its nature if it merely pursues a plan already adopted by the legislative body itself, or some power superior to it.'

2. *May Not Repeal Existing Legislation.*
   The power of direct legislation cannot be used to amend or repeal existing legislation. Thus, electors cannot compel the passage of an ordinance which is in direct conflict with a prior ordinance and which would constitute an implied repealer of that legislation. *Althouse*, supra, 255 N. W.2d at 454.
   See also *Elections #588; Ordinances and Resolutions #377, #383, #384, #388, #390, #413, and #429.*

3. **Must be Within Powers Conferred Upon Governing Body.** In initiative proceedings municipal delectors may exercise only such legislative power or authority as is conferred upon the village board or common council. *Althouse*, supra, 255 N. W. 2d at 454.
   See also Ordinances and Resolutions #401 and #427.

4. **Must Comply with Statutory Time Limits.** An initiated ordinance or resolution, even though within the ambit of the governing body's power, must be exercised under the same time schedules which bind the village board or common council. *Althouse*, supra, 255 N.W. 2d at 454.

5. **Cannot Modify Statutorily Prescribed Procedures.** If a statute prescribes set procedures, such as in the acquisition of, or additions to a public utility under sec. 66.066, 'the electors may not initiate legislation which will modify those statutorily prescribed

procedures which bind the [governing body] itself in respect to the limitations which the Wisconsin courts have placed upon direct legislation.'
Althouse, supra, 255 N. W.2d at 454;
Denning, v. City of Green Bay, 271 Wis.230, 72 N.W.2d 730 (1955)."

As can be seen by the five limitations, the electors have strong stance with regard to direct legislation. Mr. Matty's conclusions ignore number four and unfortunately by doing so, apparently felt he could misinform the council and the general public.

He apparently based his conclusions on the fact that the council passed resolution #2008-11-013, while limitation four directly states the ordinance or resolution must be exercised within the same time frames which bind the common council. As the resolution was not passed by the council until approximately one month after the petition was initiated his argument lacked any standing and only served to delay proper action by the council.

CRG membership was very disturbed by Mr. Matty's conclusion, for while his opinion conflicted with the statutes, and it could be corrected in a circuit court, the time delay could put the petition for the spring election in jeopardy. Was that the purpose of his conclusion?

An editorial by the La Crosse Tribune on December 11, 2008 again said that City Attorney Stephen Matty "argues that action taken by the council last month to set up the emergency medical services fact-finding commission conflicts under state law with a binding referendum. He said the council could choose to keep the referendum off the ballot, run it as an advisory referendum only, alter the referendum or alter the commission legislation."

He was in error and caused much wasted time and dollars by giving that opinion.

Nervousness and confusion was apparent at city hall as on December 11, 2008; the council voted overwhelmingly (15-1) to allow the measure on the ballot. A move to delete a provision that barred the council from any EMS-related actions until March when the study was to have been completed, failed after Mayor Johnsrud declined to break an 8-8 council tie.[1]

Was there an ulterior motive?

A few days later Bill Harnden called me and requested we meet to discuss the current mess. I agreed. He was of the opinion that it was time for the council to approve the petition and stop wasting time and money when it was apparent the people wanted the petition process completed and to put the ban into effect. As my intent from the beginning was only to stop the city from getting into the ambulance business, I agreed with him, and at a special council meeting on December 18, 2008 we presented a joint statement that requested the council approve the Direct Legislation and not send it to the April ballot.

As I took that position without consultation of the CRG membership, I was duly criticized for making the joint statement.

Craig Nestor a CRG member said, "I'm going to tell you something, Mr. Drewes does not represent this movement."[2]

Nestor, Dorothy Leonard and Bruce Ranis agreed the voters should have their say. Steve Gores, who at this time was considering a run against Johnsrud, also was suspicious and questioned the mayor's and Harnden's sincerity. "I think it's politically motivated because the last thing (Johnsrud) wants is this thing on the table while he's trying to run for re-election."[2]

As the city council had to make the final decision in January and as I had gotten many calls from CRG members and others in the community regarding the joint memorandum, Mr. Harden and I wrote to the council in December; I called a special CRG meeting to discuss my action. The group voted overwhelmingly to have me reflect the members desires to the council, that is, that the petition should be on the ballot in April. I did not object, as it appeared to be a win-win situation in either case. Therefore at the January 8th city council meeting I did indeed present a written statement noting the wishes of CRG, that the petition should be on the April ballot.

With all the previous discussions concerning the ability of the city to start an ambulance service, the petition's status, the city attorney's opinion, and whether or not the item should be on the April ballot, the petition should have been a rather short item on the agenda.

It took some time, but the council finally did accept the petition; therefore it will not go to the voters in April.

The council-approved study on the EMS commission was never staffed, never met and, therefore, never completed. With the results of the primary, the general election and the change in council seats, it made further study pointless.

The joint EMS commission proposed by the mediation process was intended to provide oversight and set procedures for emergency care services. The county adopted its version but while Johnsrud insisted there was agreement he would not accept the county's approved plan. The commission, as adopted by the county, determines who provides ambulance services and oversees the entire emergency medical system, including dispatch and first responders. Johnsrud wanted to limit the commission's control on both fronts.[3]

The voters speak in CAPITAL LETTERS

CRG did not take an active role in support of any of the seven candidates for mayor in the February primary. The biggest surprise was the 5th place finish for Mayor Johnsrud. Apparently the ambulance issue had made a tremendous impact on the minds of the voters, and even though the matter was settled by the city council against the wishes of many who wanted it on the ballot, it had the same effect.

The results of the primary:

Dorothy Leonard	2,431
Matt Harter	1,838
Andrea Richmond	1,011
Gary Pedesky	999
Mark Johnsrud	766
Jim Bloedorn	670
Mick Lesky	69

April 7, 2009 now became an important date for all factions, not only for those interested in the ambulance but other issues as well. Prior to the primary, Harter had certainly won the sign war as his signs were on every heavily traveled street and many off streets as well. His family was well known as they have a garbage hauling business but he was a newcomer to the political scene and only 24 years old. He had been a member of the Navy Seals but developed a physical problem and was dropped from the program.

Dorothy Leonard, his opposition, provided a great contrast in nearly every way possible. She was with Viterbo University staff and in general quite liberal. She had experience with the city government (which probably hurt her) and is, of course, female.

CRG did take a position here, as the contrast was too great to ignore. In addition, there were five city council seats open, and they also provided some interesting contrasts. We supported the following:

Mayor	Matt Harter
2nd district	Matt Harter (He ran for both)
3rd district	Chris Olson
4th district	Ron Veglahn
6th district	Mark Smith
8th district	Mary Thompson

The vote for mayor on April 7 was as follows:

Matt Harter	6,831	almost 55%
Dorothy Leonard	5,505	about 45%

As Harter was elected mayor he could not fulfill his election to the 2nd district council seat. The process in La Crosse, of filling that seat, is to have the council appoint a person who had applied to be appointed and that they felt would represent that district effectively.

Mayor Harter broke the tie of eight to eight of the council members to appoint Al Wagner to that position.

Chris Olson was successful in his bid for the 3rd district, Ron Veglahn had a very close race but came in second as did the other candidates.

CRG was proud to have been a part of the process to show that indeed,

"Yes, You Can Stop City Hall."

REFERENCES

1 LCT 12-12-2008
2 LCT 12-19-2008
3 LCT 1-10-2009

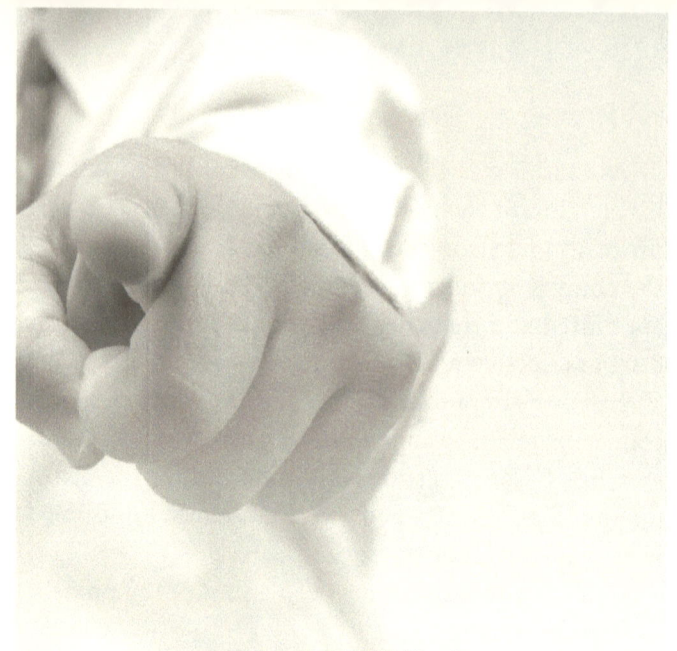

CHAPTER 6
What can you do?

There is a constant impulsion by far too many municipalities to increase the size of government and control the lives of their citizens. This is often done without the overt intent of destroying private business, but unfortunately they eventually cripple private enterprise.

Bureaucrats have a human nature, like the rest of us which seems to justify expansion of their "business" as that tends to secure their place in any organization. Certainly, the number of people under their supervision and the size of their budget assuredly will increase their status (and most likely will inflate their salaries) by showing the size of their department and how large a budget is under their control. This is a natural result that must be met with opposition by the taxpayer. Unfortunately it takes guts to take the initiative to do so.

What doesn't exist in the government sector is

the profit control that business must consider every minute of the day. The citizen voter must remind the elected officials just who is the "boss." Conversely, in business each immediate boss must always be concerned for business survival. The bureaucrat works full time, and his thoughts are in the vein of how he can show how a new or existing "service" is critical to benefit of the average citizen.

I want to note there are many government employees who do their work with great efficiency; however, that should not allow our elected officials to expand the role of government to "increase revenue" as was stated in the La Crosse push to take over the ambulance business.

It is so very important to do some homework before your local government starts to take some action to expand the number of employees they have for whatever reason. What might you do?

1. Check your state laws to see if a citizens' group can take action to start or stop an activity.

2. If there are pertinent laws, study them carefully. Your elected officials should be happy to help you understand them. In Wisconsin we have direct legislation.

3. Get to know the media in your area. They are usually nice people and in many cases are receptive to citizen input and will even agree with your point. That was the case in La Crosse.

4. Even though the item of your concern is not on the agenda of your local government, go to as many public meetings as possible. Your representative will appreciate your interest, and you will learn how the system operates.

5. Many local governments do not follow Roberts Rules very well, not because they don't want to, but because they are not much more knowledgeable than you are about parliamentary procedure.

   In fact, you may take courses in Roberts Rules and be of assistance to the group. Meet with the chair prior to a meeting and discuss the proper procedures. If you have a Toastmasters Club in your area they are often a good source of assistance. If possible seek the help of a registered parliamentarian.

6. Don't wait until the item of concern is on the agenda of the legislative body. There usually are sub committee meetings to learn of the pros and cons prior to bringing it to the floor. This takes a lot of time and work but is necessary to be effective.

7. Organize a citizens group if your community does not have one. This group should NOT be a one-issue group. It needs to be one that is concerned about good, efficient government that is open to all ideas. The group needs to press for proper compliance with open meeting laws and open records availability.

   In La Crosse we were able to recruit 76 people who worked very hard to get the required signatures for the direct legislation. We would not have been successful without them.

8. Our parent organization is located in Milwaukee, Wisconsin called Citizens for Responsible Government. They have a website, www.crgnetwork.com, and we would suggest you go there for more information. Our group in La Crosse is called CRG La Crosse County. We welcome new members who share our goals.

About the Author, David Drewes

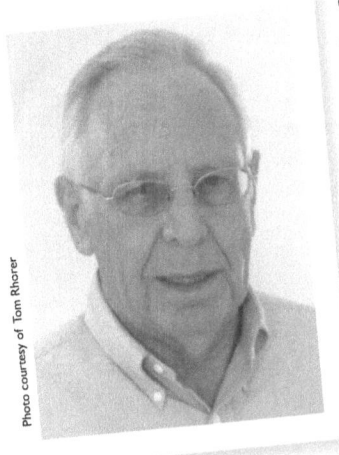

Photo courtesy of Tom Rhorer

Growing up on a farm in western Minnesota provided the basis for a conservative view of life for the author. Waste not want not was not an option but a way of life. He worked his way through college working as many as 48 hours per week yet found time to complete his degree.

The Navy gave him opportunities to learn leadership and he retired as a LCDR. His work in sales for most of his career exposed him to the knowledge of how private business will outperform government in most areas. When a group of concerned and interested parties felt there was a need for a conservative watchdog voice in the La Crosse, WI, area, they formed a local organization called "Citizens for Responsible Government La Crosse County." He was named president when it was formed in 2006 and remains the chairman to date. In addition to the successful defeat of the city's attempt to enter the ambulance business, the organization helped to convince the voters of the school district that a very expensive and in many ways wasteful bonding issue should be defeated.

He is married, has 3 children and 5 grandchildren. He is active in his church, plays golf as often as he can, and plays and teaches bridge, the greatest card game ever invented. He and his wife of more than 45 years enjoy traveling and being with the grandchildren.

www.ingramcontent.com/pod-product-compliance
Lightning Source LLC
Chambersburg PA
CBHW020356290526
45785CB00005B/2317